Heroin Death
How to Stop the Opioid Crisis

Joseph C. Mancini, MD

Cover design by Brenda Mihalko
Interior design by Sable Books

ISBN 978-1973824008

Dr. Mancini can be reached at josephcmancini@gmail.com
or (585) 645-9245 for speaking engagements or questions.

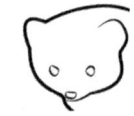

Sable Books
sablebooks.org

CONTENTS

To Janet, Chris, Annie, Julie, and Dennis for listening to me obsess about the opioid crisis for the last 15 years. And to my many opioid-dependent patients whose experiences taught me more about the crisis than any other research.

INTRODUCTION

For over ten years, I worked with many heroin addicts and people dependent on opioid pain medication. My interest in the opioid crisis and my concern for those at risk for rapid respiratory death resulting from heroin or pain pill addiction have motivated me to pursue some promising developments in this field.

To help solve the opioid crisis, I want to share some important information, so I have created a guide that will help everyone who can benefit from this knowledge to understand:

- Some of the history of opioid pain medications
- The recent rapid rise in sudden death due to opioids
- Why this class of drugs is so insidiously enticing, yet so deadly
- Strategies for decreasing opioid-related deaths

This guide deals with a very specific response to a class of drugs—opioids—that can cause up to 24% of users to become dependent on it or addicted to it (Martell et al., 2007). The opioid crisis refers to the rising number of deaths resulting from addiction. Opioid pain medications, like heroin, fall into a class of compounds that are mostly derived from opium or are chemically similar to opium.

But opium has been around for over 5000 years, so what happened? Why are so many deaths occurring now?

- In the spring of 1970, there were two deaths per month from heroin overdose. By autumn of 1970, there were two deaths per day from heroin overdose (Courtwright, 1982 and 2001).
- In 1999, there were 26 deaths per day from heroin and opioid pain pills (MMWR, 12/16/16).
- In 2014, there were 78 deaths per day from heroin and opioid pain pills, with heroin causing fewer than 50% of those (MMWR, Op. cit).
- In 2015, there were 82 deaths per day from opioids. At this time, heroin deaths surpassed death by opioid pain medication, and opioid deaths in general, surpassed deaths from gunshot wounds (Ingraham, 2006).

To stop this crisis will require widespread awareness and concerted efforts by both the public and private sectors of our society. Much is already being done by government agencies like the Centers for Disease Control and Prevention (CDC) and Food and Drug Administration (FDA), as well as professional organizations dealing with addiction. But progress also depends on the involvement of parents, teachers, coaches, employers, and health care personnel at all levels. Their awareness of any exposure their children, students, and employees may have to opioid pain medications is crucial, as is their thorough understanding of this class of drugs.

It may not be possible to prevent all deaths caused by opioids, but it is worth a try to lower the rapidly rising number of people dying from them rather than watch those numbers continue to increase.

And now there are two drugs that offer new hope. While this guide does not focus on addiction or drug overdose per se, it offers a detailed discussion of these two drugs and their ability to change the opioid crisis.

Although the treatment of psychiatric illness, addiction, or drug overdose in general may be a complex and often lifelong process, the specific nature of the opioid crisis warrants an understanding of these two drugs as a possible way to decrease the rapidly rising numbers of overdose-related deaths from opioids. Anyone affected by, or interested in, the opioid crisis stands to benefit from knowing as much as possible about these two drugs, including the reasons why the medical community and policy makers do not appreciate and promote them.

Disclaimer: I do not work for any of the companies that manufacture these two drugs.

What to expect from this guide:
Even some awareness and knowledge can help to significantly decrease what has been called the worst epidemic in United States history. So, it is my hope that this guide will provide the necessary knowledge to empower people to take action.

- It provides some background of addiction in general and opioids in particular, including a brief history of opioid development and its uses over the past five thousand years. Opioid pain medications and heroin both fall into the category of opioids, which will be explained in a later chapter.

- It explains why opioids are more addictive than any other addiction-causing substances.
- It discusses historical reasons for the epidemic of sudden deaths caused by these agents that has erupted over the past 20 years.
- It describes an opioid blocker—**naloxone**—and another unique opioid—**buprenorphine**—that is different from all others in a very critical way, to the extent that buprenorphine can now be prescribed for pain relief to prevent opioid dependence in the first place, and continue to be prescribed at a higher dose for the ongoing treatment of those already addicted to opioids.

Furthermore, this guide shows how these opioid substances have captured the imagination, political energy, and general preoccupation of humans over the last one hundred years, resulting in a marked increase in opioid use and production. While it does not deal with the complex overall management of addiction in general (or opioid addiction in particular), it does focus on the issue of **rapid respiratory death resulting from opioid addiction**—a predicament that has infiltrated all socioeconomic and educational groups, affecting people of all colors, races, and creeds.

And now there is hope—two drugs that can prevent these rising episodes of sudden death. But physicians are reluctant to use this relatively straight forward solution to a devastating problem. So, it is up to all of us—parents, teachers, employers, and health care consumers—to bring about change.

Chapter 1 — The Crisis

The type of addiction resulting from pain medication can happen to anyone, and it can happen very quickly (Lembke, 2016).

Statistics on Sudden Deaths from Opioid Pain Medications and Heroin:

Between the years 2002 and 2013, heroin-related deaths quadrupled. Between 2012 and 2013 alone, heroin-related deaths increased 39% (MMWR, 12/16/16). And in relation to that, between 1999 and 2010, prescriptions for opioid pain medications quadrupled (CDC Prescription Data, 12/20/16).

For many years, heroin was confined to inner cities and to lower socioeconomic groups. These communities often consisted of prostitutes, gamblers, thieves, adolescents from single parent homes, and jazz musicians (Courtwright, 1982 and 2001). Today, for reasons that will be explained, heroin has spread to middle and upper-class people and families in the United States. Seventy-five percent of today's heroin addicts use prescription opioid medication before they start using heroin. Ninety percent of first-time heroin users are white, have health insurance, and higher than average income (Cicero, 2014).

In relation to that, opium production in Mexico has increased 50% just in 2014 alone (Azam, 2015).

CBS News recently did a very telling story, titled "Did NFL doctors and trainers push powerful painkillers on players?" (Werner). Eighteen hundred former NFL players claimed their teams had them "popping addictive pain killers like candy to keep them from being sidelined by injuries". Former San Francisco 49ers center Jeremy Newberry was one of them, saying "Some games, I'm taking two to three Vicodin before the game, and two to three more at halftime."

Case study—first patient:
Amy was a 16-year old high school soccer player who suffered a severe sprain to her ankle during a game. She received the 'right' treatment from her primary care physician; but within a short period of time, she developed a dependence on a 'normal' prescription pain medication—Vicodin. From there, she would spiral downwards into the abuse of stronger opioids.

Due to continued pain, Amy was still being prescribed Vicodin six weeks after the injury. When she ran out of pills over a weekend, the on-call physician who didn't know her refused to refill her prescription. Because of persistent pain and early withdrawal symptoms, she convinced a friend to supply her with Vicodin and Percocet for a few days. Soon, they both ran out of pills, and Amy resorted to buying Percocet and Oxycontin on the street at very high prices.

In a later development, she learned about black tar heroin, which was cheap and worked much better and quicker. At first she snorted it, but she then learned how to inject herself—she took her first injected dose of black tar heroin on a Saturday night only one week after the on-call physician refused to prescribe medication or see her. The following morning, when her parents went to wake her up, they found her cold, blue, and not breathing.

An enticing danger:
For many people, the euphoria of opioids may be so enticing that they would gladly risk their lives. Sometimes, the downward spiral starts with an injury. Other times, it starts when people decide to experiment with opioid medications, like Vicodin, Percocet, or Oxycontin, which they may discover by chance or get from friends or relatives. For others, heroin may be their first opioid after getting high on other drugs, like alcohol, marijuana, or cocaine.

In the 1920s, 30s, and 40s, heroin was a very popular drug for jazz musicians, artists, and actors. Notable heroin fatalities include Billie Holiday, Charlie Parker, Chet Baker, Janis Joplin, and John Belushi. And just recently, the case of Philip Seymour Hoffman made headline news, an Academy Award winning actor who died of respiratory death after 25 years of sobriety. While people have been abusing opioids for the past 100 years, the rapid rise in overdose-related deaths the past 20 years has turned the situation into what is being called the worst epidemic in American history.

Case study—second patient:
The famous P. Rogers Nelson, better known as Prince (the musician and artist), died rather suddenly on April 21, 2016 at the age of 57. It has been confirmed that his death was caused by an overdose of a drug called fentanyl. Fentanyl is one of the many opioids

that can be synthesized in a laboratory; it is thus known as a synthetic opioid since it is not derived from opium itself. The drug is also 80-100 times stronger than heroin or morphine.

Prince was physically very energetic; his performances involved jumping from high stages and vigorous dancing. These strenuous activities eventually caused him to suffer severe hip pain. Prince elected not to treat this with surgery, and according to news reports began to relieve this pain with opioid pain medication.[1] A week before his death, while flying back home, his plane made an emergency landing in Illinois because he had become unresponsive, for reasons unknown. When he arrived in the emergency room, Prince was given an opioid antagonist. This immediately reversed the effects of his medication and brought him out of this unresponsiveness. Essentially, it saved Prince's life because it stopped the respiratory decline from the opioid.

A week later, apparently, Prince made trips to the drug store to get more pain medication. On April 21st, he was found dead in a home elevator. The final autopsy revealed that his death was most likely caused by fentanyl.

In both case studies—Amy and Prince—the corresponding rapid respiratory decline and sudden death suggest accidental overdose rather than suicidal overdose. That said, suicide is known to occur

---

1   The references to Prince are from the news media and are public knowledge. The author has not consulted with family for confirmation, or further details. It can be speculated that his situation was very similar to Amy's.

as a result of the extreme pain of opioid withdrawal that is often too intense to bear.

Also important to know is that accidental opioid overdose is different from other forms of accidental overdose by drugs like alcohol, hallucinogens, marijuana, or tranquilizers—in these situations, death occurs because of multiple organ damage over a longer period of time, which also allows for possible medical intervention. Rare exceptions to this are outlined in the next chapter for cocaine and methamphetamine, both being stimulants and not depressants like opioids.

CHAPTER 2 — ADDICTION IS A COMPLEX ISSUE

Addiction to mood-altering substances and habit-forming social behaviors involving food, sex, shopping, gambling, and internet use have become prevalent in our culture. In the context of addiction, drugs, food, and sex share a commonality—all three specifically stimulate a very small portion of the brain that is linked to pleasure. It is called the medial forebrain bundle and is also referred to as the pleasure pathway (Brick and Erickson, 1998). This small portion of the brain lies in the middle of the brain towards the front and is represented by a variety of nerve pathways that intermingle with one another. It is stimulated by food, sex, and drugs, as well as by many endorphin producing behaviors (Erickson, 1998).

The concept of addiction has undergone multiple changes regarding its meaning over time. Its modern definition denotes the inability to stop taking a substance. Anna Lembke, MD boils it down to three Cs: Control, Compulsion, and Consequences (Lembke, 2016). Several theories have emerged around the concept of addiction. Many believe it is a simple matter of free choice: "Just say no" (Nancy Reagan, 1980s). Others believe it is a moral failure, a weakness of character (Courtwright, 1982 and 2001). Still others suggest that addiction is related to mental health disorders in the realm of psychology (Courtwright, 1982 and 2001). For many years, several groups of people have theorized that addiction represents a true chronic disease (Erickson, 2007).

In the past 15 to 20 years, with the use of high-tech radiology tests, changes in the brains of people who are known to be addicted to a substance have been observed. In multiple research studies, there is growing evidence that addiction is a chronic condition that is no different from diseases such as diabetes, high blood pressure, cancer, and rheumatoid arthritis (Erickson, 2007). Most recently, while not denying the influence of biology and genetics, Maia Szalavitz has offered a slightly different theory that explains addiction as a learning disability (Salavitz, 2015).

Despite the varying evidence and beliefs that drive these theories, one fact is universal to them all: withdrawal from opioids stimulates an urgent need for physical relief. And one way to get relief quickly is to take more opioids that fill and satisfy the opioid receptors in the brain. In Chapter 3, the specific risk of opioid addiction, compared to all other substances, is discussed. Opioids are the only mood-altering substances that offer direct pain relief, but they also consistently and predictably cause sudden respiratory suppression that can lead to death, if enough is taken.

Endorphins: The key to understanding opioids is knowing how endorphins work—these naturally occurring substances in the brain are stimulated by pleasurable activities such as exercising, eating chocolate, drinking caffeine, watching television, using the internet, listening to music, and indulging in shopping or gambling, all of which produce feelings of euphoria, not unlike the runner's "high". Endorphins weren't discovered in the brain until 1974; their discovery has helped people understand why opioids, which have been around for over 5000 years in various forms, are so addictive. While naturally occurring endorphins can be stimulated by many things, opioids act as a substitute for endorphins and are, thus, more powerful and more dangerous.

Stimulants/relaxers: Mood-altering substances can be divided into stimulants and relaxers[1] – or uppers and downers in street talk. The best-known **stimulants** are cocaine and methamphetamine. The most common **relaxers** are opioids, alcohol, barbiturates (like phenobarbital and secobarbital), and benzodiazepines (like Valium and Xanax).

Chapter 3 explains how opioids are more complex than other drugs, thus making them much more dangerous. This is an important distinction, because the more complex opioids are primarily central nervous system **depressants or relaxers.** Opioids are substances that cause a person to feel mellow and euphoric. At the same time, in some people (roughly 20%) they can produce a mildly stimulating effect that cause this type of person to focus better (or believe that it is the case) while also feeling relaxed and mellow.[2] (See case study #3 in Chapter 5.)

---

1   Another category includes hallucinogens which alter a person's perception and thinking. These include, but are not limited to, mushrooms, LSD, and marijuana.

2   Alcohol will not be discussed even though it is also a complex substance, but in a different way from opioids. Unlike opioids, the highest risk of death from alcohol is in the withdrawal period due to the risk of seizures, which may cause death. Death does not occur during withdrawal from opioids, but only when taking a lethal dose.

Because opioids (including heroin) provide **direct pain relief**, they make users more vulnerable to addiction compared to other types of addicts. Finding a solution is, thus, also more complicated. Opioid-dependent people can be divided into several categories: those who want to stop using, those who aren't ready to stop, those who started using to get high, and those who started using inadvertently after taking a short-acting opioid to, quite appropriately, treat an acute injury. These different groups overlap and are not mutually exclusive.

CHAPTER 3 — OPIOIDS

Agonists, antagonists, and receptors:
To fully understand the opioid crisis and the need for action to prevent rapid respiratory death resulting from heroin and opioid pain medication addiction, it is useful to know more about the terms agonist, antagonist, and receptor. This chapter and Chapter 5 offer working definitions of these terms, and others, and explain their roles in both pain relief and addiction.

An **agonist** is an activator or a stimulus. It can be an internal chemical or hormone, such as an endorphin. Or, it can be an external chemical or drug, such as morphine. Agonists are either full or partial. **Full agonists** can reach their full potential if enough is given, i.e., if enough heroin is taken, it will reach its full potential and stop respirations.

Partial agonists do not reach full potential in regard to some of their effects, which will plateau and not go higher. However, the same partial agonist may have full effects in regard to other properties (see buprenorphine below).

A **receptor** is a series of amino acids and/or proteins that exist in the brain, and it attracts agonists in such a way that it becomes activated and causes a physiological response in the brain and/or body, e.g., stimulation, euphoria, sedation, hallucinations, muscle movement, or feelings.

Antagonists also bind to receptors but without any effect except for blocking other agonists (see naloxone below).

Opioids, opiates, and their relation to opium, heroin, and narcotic pain pills:

Opium is the gooey substance that exists in the pulp of the beautiful poppy seed plant—*Les Coquelicots, Papaver Somniferum* (as seen on the cover image of this guide). This gooey substance is harvested by cutting into the pulp after the flowers have dropped off. As soon as it has dried, it is available for smoking or ingestion. Opium's attraction directly relates to the euphoria generated when smoked or ingested.

Opium is an interesting substance to understand from both historical and chemical points of view. Historically, the first recorded evidence of opium appeared around 3300 B.C. on clay tablets written by the Sumerians, a tribe of people living in what is now modern-day southern Iraq (Fernandez, 1998). They made reference to a substance that gave them tremendous pleasure when ingested or smoked. For the next 5,000 years, up to 1804, opium became the center of issues relating to commercial privileges, legal and territorial concessions, international trade, illegal export, social and economic disruption due to widespread addiction, and a number of wars motivated by unequal treaties (Fernandez, 1998).

The terms opioid and opiate are often used interchangeably—here is an explanation:

Opiates: There are only three naturally occurring opiates that are extracted directly from opium: morphine, codeine, and thebaine. Morphine comprises

12% of opium. It is the most psychoactive, pain-reducing, and euphoria-producing substance of the three. It follows that the morphine component most likely accounted for the attraction to opium from 3300 B.C. to 1804 when it was harvested directly from the plant. Codeine is also a well-known pain reliever, though it is considerably weaker than morphine (see Appendix A). Thebaine provides no pain relief or euphoria, but it is the source of other semisynthetic opiates that have come into play in the current epidemic.

Semisynthetic opiates: These are opiates that are synthesized from any of the three natural opiates mentioned above. They include oxycodone (Percocet and Oxycontin), hydrocodone (Vicodin, Norco, and Lortab), hydromorphone (Dilaudid), and others.

Synthetic opiates: These are synthesized in the laboratory but are similar chemically to natural and semi-synthetic opiates and often have a more powerful effect (see Appendix A). Familiar names include fentanyl, carfentanil, and methadone.

Morphine is a natural opiate that was extracted from opium in 1804. Codeine was extracted from opium in 1832. Heroin, a semisynthetic opioid was synthesized from morphine in 1874, though it was not released onto the market until 1898. Bayer Pharmaceuticals originally released what was thought to be a non-addictive, heroin-based cough suppressant that was sold over-the-counter. Ironically, also in 1898, aspirin was a prescription medication and, therefore, not available over-the-counter (Fernandez, 1998). When the addictive quality of heroin was discovered, legislation surrounding opioids was introduced. Over the next century, heroin use would wax and wane.

Some commonly known brand names:
The following brands are important because they are well-known to both addicts and pain patients, and many of them are easily available 'on the street' at a very high price.

In 1917, oxycodone was developed. Then laboratories developed **Percocet**, containing the primary component oxycodone combined with acetaminophen (Tylenol). Next, laboratories developed **Oxycontin**, which is oxycodone combined with other chemicals that allows it to last up to 12 hours in the blood rather than the usual four hours.

Oxymorphone was then synthesized, which is twice as strong as oxycodone. It is the main ingredient in **Opana**; like Oxycontin, it can remain in the blood for up to 12 hours.

In 1920, hydrocodone was developed from codeine. Hydrocodone is six times stronger than codeine but weaker than oxycodone (Appendix A). Hydrocodone became the main ingredient in **Vicodin**,[1] **Norco** and **Lortab**, which are all combinations of hydrocodone and acetaminophen (Tylenol).

In 1924, hydromorphone (**Dilaudid**) was synthesized from morphine; it is almost five times stronger than morphine (see Appendix A).

In 1937, **methadone** was synthesized; it is a syn-

---

1   In 2013, Vicodin was the most frequently prescribed medication in America above all other drugs of all classes.

thetic opioid that is made in a laboratory, and is commonly prescribed for the treatment of both addiction and pain.

This was followed in 1960 by **fentanyl** (the drug that killed Prince). **This is important to know: fentanyl is 80 to 100 times stronger than morphine and has been implicated in the increasing number of overdose-related deaths**. Not only is fentanyl sold on the black market but it has been found in many batches of heroin (Nelson, 2016).

In 1961, the very important discovery of naloxone occurred. This substance may be better known by its brand name: **Narcan**—the unique feature of naloxone is that it provides no pain relief but is a complete opioid blocker. Naloxone is the rescue drug that is now being given at the scene of an overdose to save the life of the opioid victim, if properly administered within minutes of respiratory arrest. **Also important to know: naloxone is a crucial part of the rescue strategies offered in this guide, because it stops the respiratory suppression caused by all full agonist opioids.** Police officers around the country are being trained to use naloxone. In April, 2017, New Mexico recently became the first state to require that its officers learn how to administer it into the nose or by injection.

In 1974, a substance called **carfentanil** was synthesized; it is 10,000 times stronger than morphine and, therefore, 100 times stronger than fentanyl. It was found in a batch of heroin in Cincinnati in September of 2016 after it caused nine deaths within nine days (NYTimes, 9/5/16).

In 1978, came the breakthrough drug **buprenorphine**—it will be discussed at length in Chapter 5, because it is a crucial part of the proposed rescue strategies.

It is important to understand why opioids are so addictive:

1. Opioids are the only mood-altering substances that give direct pain relief.
2. Opioids provide an intense degree of euphoria that has been described as transcendent by many users.
3. Opioids cause extremely painful and intense withdrawal symptoms, which make it very difficult not to seek another dose to get relief, thus fueling the vicious addictive cycle.

The National Survey on Drug Use and Health (NS-DUH) from the National Institute of Mental Health (NIH) estimated that in 2015 there were 6.2% of adults age 18 and older with Alcohol Use Disorder (AUD). Teenagers between ages 12 and 17 had a 2.5% prevalence rate.

In contrast, a meta-analysis of five studies on opioid use for low back pain showed that up to 24% of candidates indicated aberrant medicating behaviors (Martell et al., 2007). They also found that the lifetime substance use disorders in this population ranged from 36% to 56%, and the estimates of current substance use disorders were as high as 43%.

The National Safety Council recently surveyed 500 companies with over 50 employees and found that more than 70% of these companies were impacted by prescription drug misuse.

The consequences of opioid abuse:
The distinguishing, and most frightening, consequence of opioid addiction compared to other mood-altering substances is potential rapid respiratory death. There is only a brief moment between loss of consciousness and **respiratory drive decline** when too much is taken. What makes this outcome so highly probable is that a person can be taking increasing amounts of opioids and continue to feel the desire and urge to take even more, until the rapid and fatal point that breathing stops (Erickson, 2007). The one, fortunate, exception is buprenorphine.

The consequences of abusing other mood-altering substances, like alcohol, barbiturates, or benzodiazepines (Valium, Xanax, Ativan) differ significantly from the potentially fatal danger of overdosing on opioids. The first sign of overdose would be loss of consciousness; since these substances affect many systems of the body, death may occur due to multiple body organ damage over a period of time, sometimes allowing medical treatment to prolong a person's life, often with good long-term outcome. Rare exceptions to this are arrhythmias (electrical malfunction) of the heart caused by cocaine and methamphetamine (Erickson, 2007).

Sudden death caused by a stimulant is rare and idiosyncratic, whereas full agonist (stimulator) opioids will always cause respiratory suppression and death if a high enough amount is taken. The ability of opioids to consistently and predictably shut down the respiratory drive is the reason we are now in the midst of this epidemic of sudden death caused by opioids, both from heroin and opioid pain medications.

The antidote to sudden respiratory suppression: An important concept to understand is **affinity** (Budd & Raffa, 2005). Affinity refers to an opioid's ability to attach itself to the brain, similar to the pull of a magnet. Both naloxone and buprenorphine have a strong affinity for opioid receptors—this means if either one of these substances is already in the brain, it will block another opioid by preventing it from attaching itself to the brain. Conversely, if another opioid is already in the brain and causing pain relief, euphoria, or respiratory arrest, the introduction of naloxone or a large enough dose of buprenorphine will bump that opioid off the receptor and allow the person to breathe again. Because naloxone works faster than buprenorphine, it is the primary drug of choice in a respiratory arrest situation. Buprenorphine has become more useful in stopping withdrawal symptoms because it attaches itself quickly to the brain which is in need of relief, and in so doing, stops withdrawal without causing a high.

Naloxone—the rescue drug

Naloxone (Narcan) is an opioid blocker, the CPR for opioid overdose and respiratory failure. It can displace a deadly opioid from the brain and render it ineffective, thus allowing the person to spontaneously start breathing again.

Timing, however, is a crucial requirement as it must be given as soon as possible after the person has stopped breathing. The logistics can be daunting: like CPR or AED machines that reverse fatal cardiac arrhythmias, naloxone must be available at the right time, in the right place, and in the hands of a knowledgeable person.

Naloxone has been used in emergency rooms for decades on unresponsive patients. And now, to stop overdose-related deaths, big strides are being made in making it available and training medical personnel as well as lay people on how to administer it (see Resources). Some police departments around the country are receiving training since they are often the first ones on the scene (Huffington Post, 12/19/16). But this is not enough. Parents who have children dependent on heroin or pain medication should have naloxone at their disposal and know how to administer it. This also applies to teachers and coaches, who often do not know that a student is on opioids until respirations stop. Employers must be aware of the risk too, and be prepared to administer naloxone when needed (Lopez, G. Surgeon General report, Vox, 4/5/18). Remember, if naloxone is given to someone who has stopped breathing for a reason other than opioid overdose, it can cause **no** harm.

Like CPR and AED defibrillators, which are now more available in public places, naloxone needs more exposure (see Resources). The ultimate solution rests upon the knowledge and availability of buprenorphine as well as naloxone (see Chapter 6).

The impact of legislation and politics on opioid management:
Throughout the 20th century, legislation and politics have played a big role in both the supply and demand of narcotics, and they have continued to do so up to the current situation. What follows is some political background explaining why buprenorphine is underutilized and misunderstood,

particularly by practicing physicians and other health care providers.

Since 1900 there have been no fewer than ten pieces of legislation or amendments to legislation related to the topic of heroin and opioids in general (Courtwright, 1982 and 2001). Five of these are the most relevant to this discussion, of which two are crucial. In summary, from 1804 (when morphine was extracted from opium) until 1906—eight years after heroin was released—there was essentially no legislation related to opioids. However, it soon became obvious that heroin was addictive and the first piece of legislation addressing the issue was the **Pure Food and Drug Act**, approved in 1906 (Courtwright, 1982 and 2001). This Act required labeling of all opioid-based products containing heroin or morphine to alert consumers that these substances had been added to certain pharmaceutical preparations, both over the counter[2] and by prescription.

The next important piece of legislation was the **Harrison Narcotics Act** in 1914 (Courtwright, 1982 and 2001), which made it illegal to use morphine to treat opioid addicts. This meant that an addict could not be put on morphine as a form of maintenance treatment. Physicians were allowed to prescribe morphine for 'legitimate medical reasons only'. Unfortunately, this Act set the tone for the next 50 years during which any form of opioid maintenance was illegal. With the introduction of methadone in the mid-to-late sixties, the maintenance restriction was lifted by way of calling the entire methadone project a research trial and demonstration project. Chapter 5 contains further details about methadone.

---

2   For example, paregoric for colicky babies is opioid based.

In 1970, the **Controlled Substance Act** (Courtwright, 1982 and 2001) was passed. Set up by the Drug Enforcement Administration (DEA), it created schedules of drugs ranging from Schedule I to Schedule V. The DEA placed all the illegal drugs such as heroin into Schedule I. Schedule II was for prescription opioids and other habit-forming medications that did not allow physicians to write refills. Schedule III contained slightly less addictive preparations that did allow refills. Schedules IV and V are all other medications that have very slight but possible risk for dependency.

The last two pieces of legislation are the most important. In 2000, the Drug Addiction Treatment Act, **DATA 2000** (TIP 40 pgs. 79-85) was passed. The goal was to allow physicians with special training to prescribe the drug buprenorphine from their offices as a form of withdrawal treatment and for opioid maintenance, i.e.: as a substitute for heroin and other full opioids instead of methadone, which had by then become the mainstay of opioid replacement therapy and required dispensing from federally qualified treatment centers. Methadone use contained significant risks and many logistical issues.

Unlike buprenorphine, methadone[3] can cause respiratory death as well as a significant degree of euphoria if enough is taken. It also does not block other opioids the way buprenorphine does, so someone on methadone can take heroin and still overdose.

---

3   Methadone did and still does require dispensation from a federally certified clinic in which opioid-dependent people pick up and consume their daily dose in the presence of a trained addiction worker so as not to divert or misuse the drug.

Two very important aspects of DATA 2000 need further explanation. First, in order for a physician to prescribe buprenorphine, an eight hour certification course and a special DEA registration number were required. Second, the bill restricted the physician to a total of 30 patients on buprenorphine. By 2003, within two years of its release, it had become obvious that access to buprenorphine was very limited. At that point, the official limit was raised to 100 patients per physician. It is also noteworthy that only physicians, not physician assistants (PAs) or nurse practitioners (NPs), were allowed to take the certification course and prescribe the medication.

The most recent legislation was signed into law by then President Obama, called the Comprehensive Addiction and Recovery Act (**CARA**)[4] in July of 2016 (NYTimes, 7/13/16, Huettman & Emmarie). CARA primarily expanded the number of patients a doctor could treat with buprenorphine from 100 to 275. Another important change allows NPs and PAs to become certified. These specific changes were a small part of this comprehensive bill, which addressed issues of addiction in the areas of prevention, treatment, recovery, law enforcement, and criminal justice reform.

---

4   This law applies to other mood-altering substances as well as opioids.

CHAPTER 4 — THE OPIOID CRISIS, WHY NOW?

Since opium has been around for at least 5000 years, morphine for at least 200 years, and heroin for over a century, how do we explain the exponential rise in sudden deaths from this family of compounds over the last twenty years? Three very significant phenomena occurred almost simultaneously over the past 30 years that may explain the nature of, and provide possible solutions to, this epidemic.

Phenomenon #1:
During the 1970s, there were strong opinions that terminal cancer patients were being under-treated for pain. In England, a nurse named Cicely Saunders led the way to the hospice movement. In the context of terminally ill patients receiving inadequate pain medication, opioids became the new approach to hospice care to ensure these patients would be comfortable at their end stage of life (Quinones, 2015). As this became generally more acceptable, the feeling in the United States during the 1980s was that opioids could also benefit people with non-cancer chronic pain, like arthritis, low back pain, and chronic headaches without the risk for addiction (Quinones, 2015).

Two critical publications in the 1980s essentially set the stage for the epidemic that began in the

1990s. The first publication was issued by a Boston University physician, named Hershel Jick, MD. Dr. Jick was commissioned to build a database of the effects of drugs used in hospitals.[1] During his work in the late 1970s, the database grew to a sizable 300,000 patients. His assignment was to look at every drug hospitalized patients were given and to correlate them with any side effects. Dr. Jick and his research assistant, Jane Porter, specifically focused on 12,000 hospitalized patients who had been given at least one opioid medication while in the hospital in 1979. Surprisingly, they found that only four of the 12,000 patients had become addicted. But the fact that no further information was taken into account regarding duration or dose of treatment made this work merely a superficial observation and not a reliable study of any kind. Nevertheless, they communicated their finding to the editor of the New England Journal of Medicine in a letter entitled "Addiction rare in patients treated with narcotics" (Quinones, 2015). The gist of their disclosure read, "of almost 12,000 patients treated with opiates while in the hospital before 1979, only four had grown addicted." It simply cited the numbers and made no claim beyond that.

The reason this inconsequential finding became so influential was that a well-known pain specialist, Russell Portenoy, MD, was working at Sloan-Kettering Hospital in New York in 1986. Based on Dr. Jick›s letter, he decided to look at 38 of his patients and discovered that only two chronic pain sufferers had become addicted to opioids. Additionally, he noted that each of them had a history of drug abuse. He wrote an article, the second influential

---

1   This came out of the thalidomide scandal of 1960.

publication, in the journal, *Pain*, referencing Dr. Jick's letter from 1980 and concluding that opioids were not inherently addictive (Portenoy et al, 1986). Thanks to his work, Dr. Portenoy and other thought leaders concluded that any addiction pointed to the patient rather than the drug; and when they realized there may be a stigma attached to opioid prescribing, they started an effort to remove this stigma (Quinones, 2015 & PROP website, Portenoy video).

The eventual belief in opioids not being addictive in combination with the idea of noncancerous pain being under-treated constituted the first part of the "why now?" Ironically, recent research has shown that long term use of opioids for chronic pain can possibly make the pain worse (Servick, 2016).

Phenomenon #2:
In 1996, Purdue Pharmaceuticals released the well-known drug Oxycontin. The company started a campaign to convince physicians that the drug was non-addictive, based on the simple belief held by pain specialists that it was not. They further tried to convince physicians that even if Oxycontin were addictive, it was less addictive than short-acting forms of opioids since it was a form of slow-release medication lasting over 10 to 12 hours; therefore, it did not provide a short spike in blood levels and potential buzz that short-acting forms of oxycodone, hydrocodone, or other opioids provided.

Purdue Pharmaceuticals proceeded to train its drug representatives to bombard physicians (mostly at primary care offices) with this concept. Based on the publications by Dr. Jick, Ms. Porter, and Dr. Portenoy, they preached the sentiment that the long-acting property was less addictive and that opioids in general were not very addictive. They told doctors there was literature to back up this claim but did not supply any references. It is worth remembering that neither publication resembled a controlled research study. There is also evidence that Purdue Pharmaceuticals knew that opioids were inherently addictive and specifically trained their representatives to teach the opposite. It is probably no coincidence that this latter allegation led to the settlement of a federal lawsuit in 2005. To avoid prison sentences for its executives—Purdue Pharmaceuticals paid a $634.5 million fine, of which $34 million was paid by Chief Executive Officer Michael Friedman, General Counsel Howard Udell, and Chief Medical Officer Paul Goldenheim. They were each given three years probation and 400 hours of community service (Quinones, 2015).

Two parts of "The Why Now" are now in place to set the stage for the pending painkiller epidemic: the first being the false belief that opioids were intrinsically not addictive, and the second that Purdue Pharmaceuticals misbranded and misrepresented the addictive potential of Oxycontin.[2]

Phenomenon #3

This development would form the cornerstone of the rising overdose-related deaths over the past

---

2 To the credit of Dr. Portenoy, in 2013 he admitted that if he "knew then what he knew now," he would not have taught his belief of the non-addictive properties of opioids. He acknowledged that he was trying to de-stigmatize opioid prescribing, and he admitted his claims had been inappropriately based on the Jick letter and his own survey of only 38 patients. Dr. Portenoy remains a well-respected member of the pain community and should be commended on his openness and honesty about his baseless contributions to this tremendous epidemic (Physicians for Responsible Opioid Prescribing, Website).

decade. A black tar heroin grower and distribution movement originated in a small town named Xalisco, Mexico. Xalisco is located in the state of Nayarit on the western Mexican coast, not far from Puerto Vallarta. The city of Xalisco has a mere 21,800 people. This small town is important because by the mid-nineties the sugarcane farmers had set up a very efficient delivery system of black tar heroin to over a dozen major areas in the western United States. In the late 90s, this distribution enterprise expanded east of the Mississippi River. These sugarcane farmers changed their crop from sugarcane to poppy seed plants that yielded vast amounts of opium. They then synthesized an inexpensive but powerful form of heroin from the opium that they were growing (Quinones,2015).

Here is how it worked. Farmers living in Xalisco created franchises (or heroin cells), and these franchise owners hired operators who lived in the United States. The operators received telephone orders for black tar heroin, which franchise owners smuggled into the United States, while also illegally transporting young males across the border to become drivers. These drivers were paid a weekly wage, room and board, and were given a car. Their income was not dependent on how much they delivered, thus eliminating a motive for cutting the heroin with something to make a greater profit. Because black tar heroin tends to be pure, it is very powerful. The drivers placed the heroin into balloons, which they hid in their mouths while making their deliveries.[3] They were known to

---

3   In his 2015 book, *Dreamland*, Sam Quinones reported that an informant in Denver in the mid-90s estimated that a single driver could expect to gross $5,000 per day almost immediately and up to $15,000 daily after the first year.

transport up to 30 balloons at a time, looking like 'chipmunks' driving around town (Quinones, Op. cit.). Should a driver be stopped by the police, they could quickly swallow the balloons to avoid arrest, and hopefully not die from the enormous amount of heroin in their stomachs (unless a balloon broke, of course).

As for the unknowing users who switched from narcotic pain medication to black tar heroin, they really had no idea what dose they were taking. And this gullibility has contributed to the staggering number of accidental overdose deaths, as in the first case study patient, Amy.

Chapter 5 — Buprenorphine, The Only Safe Opioid

It is clear how the aforesaid three phenomena culminated in the current epidemic of rapid respiratory deaths from opioid overdose. This paints a picture of why in the past 20 years, heroin has gone from an inner city drug associated with low-income people and jazz musicians to middle and upper middle class people of all kinds.

At this point, it is appropriate to ask **what now?** How can this epidemic be stopped? For many people, heroin use resulted from a desire to get high, often after using other mood altering substances. But recent statistics indicate that 75% of people currently on heroin were taking narcotic pain pills first (as in the case of Amy), before switching to heroin, which has now surpassed pain medications as the cause for sudden opioid death (Cicero, 2014). While pain medication is usually appropriately prescribed for relief from acute pain, people are increasingly using these drugs for the sole purpose of getting high. It is now being reported that long term use of opioids can actually make chronic pain worse, as noted previously (Servick, 2016).

It has yet to be determined through research what percentage of people on opioid pain medication obtained it by legal prescription to treat a genuine condition, like an acute injury or after surgery, versus obtaining it illegally to feed their addiction. Be that as it may, according to Martell (2007), in the first group alone many people will benefit from appropriate use of buprenorphine, i.e., up to 24% of whom demonstrate aberrant drug taking behaviors and up to 56% of whom have substance use disorders.

Buprenorphine—the only safe opioid:
What is buprenorphine? And how will it protect the above mentioned group of people and, ultimately, decrease the number of people dying from heroin and pain medications?

A unique drug: To understand the distinct mechanism of buprenorphine, it will help to review the first part of Chapter 3 that refers to agonists and antagonists, specifically agonist opioids and their ability to attach to the brain until respiration stops. So then, what makes buprenorphine unique? It is a partial agonist (stimulator) in terms of respiratory depression, possibly due to its inherent agonist-antagonist properties (Jasinski, 1978), i.e., it has a limited effect regarding respiration and degree of euphoria, but it has a fuller effect for pain relief (see discussion below).

History: The history of buprenorphine, the politics around it, and the legislation affecting it, have contributed to its under-utilization in the treatment of pain and addiction. Research at the U.S. federal prison and psychiatric hospital in Lexington, KY (often referred to as 'The Narcotics Farm') between 1935 and 1964, as well as the work of chemist John W. Lewis, Ph.D at Reckitt-Coleman, Inc. in England in the 60s—a search for an opioid with the benefits of morphine but not the side effects—resulted in the synthesis of buprenorphine in 1969.

Buprenorphine is a unique opioid that acts as a very effective pain medication. From 1981 until the early 2000s, anesthesiologists used buprenorphine in intravenous and subcutaneous forms, primarily as an adjunct to surgical anesthesia and postoperative pain relief. Buprenorphine is most effective intravenously or subcutaneously (under the skin), as well as sublingually (placed under the tongue or on the inside of the cheek, known as the buccal area), where it gets absorbed immediately without having to pass through the gastrointestinal tract. If ingested, the majority of it gets neutralized in the stomach.

Safety properties of buprenorphine—ceiling effect: Unlike all other opioids, buprenorphine has a natural cut-off for some of its effects. Instead of rising, some effects level off no matter how high a dose is taken. The ceiling effect occurs because it is a partial rather than a full agonist, and has antagonist as well as agonist properties.

An effective pain reliever: Essentially, buprenorphine works as a partial stimulator in regards to respiratory depression and euphoria, but is a full agonist for analgesia (Dahan, 2006). Buprenorphine is 30 times stronger than morphine (see Appendix B for morphine equivalents). The key to its use for pain relief in relation to respiratory depression is found in animal studies. Buprenorphine's ceiling effect for respiratory depression is thought to be around 0.1 mg per kg, whereas the ceiling for pain control is closer to somewhere between 1 and 3 mg per kg (Cowan, 1977). One clinical human study shows some indication that although there is a ceiling effect for respiratory depression, there may not be a ceiling effect at all for pain relief

(Budd & Collett, 2003). This gives buprenorphine the unique potential as a pain reliever without the risk of respiratory depression and consequent death, in contrast to morphine and all the other full agonists. As for its effectiveness in chronic pain control, Daitch et al (2014) reported reduced pain scores and improved quality of life scores for 35 chronic pain patients who were converted from high dose full-opioid agonists to sublingual buprenorphine.

The use of buprenorphine in the United States: Starting in the mid 1990s, sublingual buprenorphine was being prescribed in France at higher doses for the treatment of addiction to opioids. When the FDA investigated it for use in the U.S., they found two reported cases of sudden death resulting from very high doses of buprenorphine combined with high doses of a benzodiazepine (Valium, Xanax) injected intravenously. Because of these two cases, the FDA did not approve buprenorphine until it was combined with naloxone. This may sound counter-intuitive, and the use of an antagonist for treating addiction has caused much confusion. But the FDA insisted on this combination because of attempts by people in France to use buprenorphine for getting high; even though it causes very little euphoria, injection attempts were made. That being said, only when it was combined with a high dose of a depressant like Valium, did death occur. Naloxone is virtually inert if taken under the tongue, but will precipitate acute withdrawal if injected, hence the attempt by the U.S. to discourage injection.

In addition to generic buprenorphine-naloxone combination tablets for sublingual use, it is currently available in a buccal film form under the brand names Bunavail, Suboxone, and Zubsolv. Although the presence of naloxone is a safety feature in the higher dose preparations to discourage injection of the drug, the ultimate reason for its low risk is the ceiling effect mentioned above, which is an intrinsic quality of buprenorphine.

Further safety studies: Besides the animal studies and the theoretical reasons for the respiratory safety of buprenorphine due to the ceiling effect, several autopsy studies have indicated the rarity of buprenorphine alone causing death. One study showed that "of the 98 overdose fatalities studied in NYC in 2013, only two tested positive for buprenorphine metabolites" and both involved multiple substances (Paone, 2015).

It is important to be aware of the similarities and differences between buprenorphine and methadone, since both are used in the treatment of pain as well as addiction. While both are long acting and can satisfy the opioid receptor, methadone has no ceiling effect, thus making it exponentially riskier for accidental overdose and consequent respiratory death. **Methadone** has been useful since the early 70s to treat opioid addiction because of its long-acting property; but due to its significant risk, it continues to be dispensed under very strict guidelines in federally qualified clinics rather than from a doctor's office as in the case of buprenorphine-naloxone combined or buprenorphine alone. Two characteristics of **buprenorphine** help it to stop withdrawal symptoms within 20 minutes while providing rapid relief: its tight affinity (attaching to the brain and blocking other opioids) and its partial stimulating effects (not causing the person to become high but satisfying the brain sufficiently to induce a sense of comfort often described as 'feeling normal').

Case study—third patient: Rhonda's story took place before 2003 when buprenorphine was not yet available in the sublingual form for the treatment of opioid dependence. She is a Ph.D. biochemist who worked in opioid research. Suffering chronic back pain, and due to multiple surgeries, she was prescribed Oxycontin by her physician. She not only got pain relief and experienced some euphoria, but also felt energized and more focused. Rhonda realized she had a problem when she spent an entire night typing a research paper, finally finishing around 6:00 a.m., before going to sleep. When she awoke several hours later, she discovered she had actually typed the same paragraph repeatedly about 30 times instead of the whole paper. At that point, Rhonda also went into a painful withdrawal, and realized she had two options to relieve her symptoms: increase her Oxycontin dose, or take buprenorphine.

Rhonda went to an emergency room and requested buprenorphine. The physician had no idea what she was talking about. After informing him about its benefits, he agreed to administer it, and her withdrawal symptoms resolved within 20 minutes. Rhonda soon realized that she had developed a craving for opioids for more reasons than just relieving her chronic pain. At that time, buprenorphine was only available in injectable form. Fortunately, she was able to find an addiction specialist who treated her accordingly to diminish her cravings. When the sublingual form became available, she was able to manage her opioid dependency together with her primary care physician and control her pain at the same time.[1]

Resistance by physicians to prescribe buprenorphine:
When buprenorphine became available in 2003, the federal government instituted two prescription requirements for the treatment of addiction, essentially to prevent abuse and sudden withdrawal if given too early:

- an 8-hour certification course[2]
- a special DEA registration number

Of the nearly 1 million physicians throughout this country, fewer than 20,000 have become certified to prescribe buprenorphine, while fewer than 5,000 are actually prescribing the medication (Stein, 2016). As difficult as it was to eliminate the stigma from using opioids in the first place, it has become even more difficult to dispel the myth that this medication is too complex to prescribe.

A number of reasons explain the unwillingness of physicians to prescribe buprenorphine:

1. The eight-hour course for proper certification and extra paperwork to get the special DEA number seem to deter many physicians.
2. There seems to be an impression that this specific certification may attract heroin addicts

---

1   Patients # 1 and 3 are fictionalized versions of actual patients known to the author.
2   The federal requirement of extra training to prescribe a particular type of medication has never been asked of any other drug produced in this country.

to their offices, while they forget that 10%–20% of their current patients are probably already dependent on opioids—those who have either developed tolerance (requiring higher and higher doses for the same effect) or are abusing them. Recent studies (as noted above) show that long-term use of most opioids for noncancerous pain either stop working or make the pain worse, though this last phenomenon is much less pronounced for buprenorphine (Pergolizzi, 2010).

3. There seems to be an impression that the eight-hour course requirement was motivated by risks and/or difficulties involved in prescribing buprenorphine.

4. To the above mentioned point, the actual reasons for the course were two-fold: (a) the FDA did not want 'pill mills' developing around the country (b) because the dose for addiction treatment was on the high side, the timing of **the first dose** (only) was important. If the first dose is given while another full agonist is in a person's system (and before that person actually goes into withdrawal), buprenorphine will bump it off the receptor and take its place (due to its strong affinity). Because buprenorphine does not have the same full effect, the person will feel a sudden drop in opioid effect and experience sudden withdrawal. In contrast, if the first dose is given when the person is already in withdrawal, it will create rapid relief from the withdrawal symptoms because it is strong enough to satisfy the receptor (which is in need of opioid support, to which it had become accustomed). This concept can be taught in a simple one-hour lecture, as is common for many other new drugs on the market.

The most recent form of buprenorphine to be approved by the FDA is crucial to the proposed solution to the opioid crisis. In October 2016, the FDA approved a lower dose buccal buprenorphine product—a film form that is placed inside the mouth (similar to Bunavail, Suboxone, and Zubsolv)—that is directly absorbed into the bloodstream. The difference is that it comes in low doses, and is approved for pain relief, not the treatment of addiction. Furthermore, it can be prescribed by any physician, PA, or NP without the eight-hour certification course and special DEA number requirement. In other words, if providers can prescribe any other opioid (Oxycontin, Percocet, Vicodin) from Schedule II, they can now prescribe this form of buprenorphine that is in Schedule III, where less addictive drugs are placed. And just to reiterate: it is very effective for pain relief, without the risk of addiction or consequent overdose-related death.

In addition, in this low dose form, buccal buprenorphine does not precipitate sudden withdrawal if given too early while a full agonist is still in the system. In fact, it has been shown that in the low analgesic dose range, buprenorphine can have a **positive additional** effect when combined with a full agonist, no matter in which order they are given (Tallarida, 2000). The additive value of morphine for episodic breakthrough pain in patients receiving low-dose buprenorphine has also been demonstrated (Mercadante, 2006). In other words, a low dose does not block full agonists the way a high dose does, and a low dose will not cause withdrawal if a full agonist is in a person's system, the way a high dose will. So, whether a high dose is used for the treatment of addiction (requiring the eight-hour course) or a low dose is used for pain treatment (not requiring the course), in both instances buprenorphine is extremely effective.

BUPRENORPHINE
1. Minimal or no withdrawal symptoms
2. Cannot cause overdose death at any dose when taken alone
3. 30X stronger than morphine for pain relief

ALL OTHER OPIOIDS
1. Severe, painful withdrawal symptoms
2. Respiratory suppression and death when a high enough dose is taken
3. Effective pain relief varies from opioid to opioid (Appendix A)

Chapter 6 — Strategies to Stop The Crisis

In the preceding chapters, this guide has given an overview of the history of opioid pain medications, the recent rapid rise in sudden death due to opioids, the attraction and dangers of this class of drugs, and strategies for treating pain without the same risk of addiction as well as decreasing overdose-related deaths by using the opioid blocker naloxone and partial agonist buprenorphine.

It cannot be stressed enough that widespread awareness and concerted efforts by both the public and private sectors of our society are needed to stop the opioid crisis. Here is a summary of the most important opportunities for intervention:

1. When someone who has been put on a three-to-ten-day course of a short-acting opioid like Vicodin or Percocet for pain relief from injury or surgery feels longer pain relief is required, and stronger than acetaminophen or ibuprofen is needed for the pain, then low-dose buccal buprenorphine can be considered.
2. When someone is chronically opioid dependent, aggressive and comprehensive treatment is needed. In addition to formal substance abuse treatment or 12 step work, what is known as "Medication Assisted Treatment" must be offered. In addition to buprenorphine which is covered in detail in chapter

5, two other drugs are available to support the opioid addict and improve chances for successful recovery and decrease the risk of sudden death. These are methadone and naltrexone. (Lopez, G. Vox 11/15/17). Like buprenorphine, methadone decreases craving and stabilizes opioid receptors. It is more risky than buprenorphine, and must be dispensed in federally qualified treatment centers. Naltrexone is a long acting form of naloxone that is a blocker and prevents overdose. It does little for craving however, but can be helpful for the highly motivated person.

3. When respirations stop, Naloxone is the rescue drug that can be given at the scene of an overdose to save the life of the opioid victim.

Additional strategies involve all of society:
Parents, teachers, coaches, counselors, and employers must educate themselves about opioids and heighten their vigilance toward children, students, athletes, and employees. But there are several things that must occur in addition to the specific actions that these role players can take:

- Awareness and access to Naloxone must reach the level that CPR and AEDs have reached in this country (see Resources under NIDA website, Samhsa, and *The Atlantic* article for more information about Naloxone). In April of 2017, New Mexico became the first state to require police officers to have access, and know how, to administer Naloxone. Citizens can, and should, lobby their state legislators to do the same.
- Increased access to high-dose buprenorphine-naloxone combination (Bunavail, Suboxone, Zubsolv, and generic forms), to be used in

conjunction with comprehensive addiction treatment for those already addicted (NAABT). This requires increased funding for addiction treatment, as well as criminal justice reform so that non-violent drug offenders who are addicted are offered treatment programs rather than incarceration.

- Increased awareness of low-dose buccal buprenorphine (Belbuca) for the treatment of pain in order to prevent the downward spiral from even starting in the first place, as in the cases of our three patients. Much like it took Dr. Portenoy and many pain specialists to de-stigmatize the prescribing of opioids for cancer and non-cancer pain in the 80s and 90s, it will take a similar or even more aggressive effort by the medical community to de-stigmatize and demystify the prescribing of both low-dose and high-dose buprenorphine for the treatment of pain and addiction. The CDC has already taken a first step by publishing 12 recommendations to help clinicians prescribe an optimal and safe course of treatment for pain (Dowell & Campos-Outcalt, 2016). While this is a good first start, it is not enough—the prescription opioids are streaming out of physician practices and the black tar heroin is pouring in from Xalisco as well as from other places.

- The FDA must approve low-dose buccal buprenorphine for the treatment of acute as well as chronic pain, for which it is now approved. It's use for acute pain has a long history since 1981 when it was approved for post operative pain, which by definition is acute pain. Pergolizzi et al, (2016) showed that low-dose buccal buprenorphine works for chronic low-back pain. By approving it for acute pain, doctors, nurse practitioners, and physician assistants would then have the option to prescribe it immediately for an acute injury, and not be forced to use hydrocodone (Vicodin), oxycodone (Percocet), or hydromorphone (Dilaudid) before switching to buprenorphine if more opioids are considered necessary.

So, what exactly can these various role players know and do to decrease the rate of sudden death from heroin and narcotic pain medications? Reading *Dreamland* by Sam Quinones and *Drug Dealer, MD: How Doctors Were Duped, Patients Got Hooked, and Why It's So Hard to Stop* by Anna Lembke, MD. will provide a more thorough background and understanding of the opioid crisis.

Furthermore:

1. All groups must be aware that addiction is a complex, lifelong affliction that requires many resources: from medication assisted treatment (MAT) to psychotherapy to 12-step work, for the rest of the person's life with the risk of relapse always looming (Philip Seymour Hoffman died a rapid respiratory death from an opioid overdose after 25 years of sobriety). Additional resources (i.e. a holistic approach), like yoga, yoga therapy, acupuncture, hypnotism, cognitive behavioral therapy (CBT), emotional behavioral therapy (EBT), exercise and nutrition must all be considered for the person suffering from addiction.

2. Employers have a very specific challenge, and clear mandate by the National Safety Council

Survey, to identify workers who are misusing pain medication and, thus, at risk for overdose. Besides 70% of these companies recognizing the problem, 75% of them do not offer training on how to deal with it, and 41% of those companies who do drug testing, do not test for synthetic or semisynthetic opioids like fentanyl, hydrocodone, and oxycodone.

3. It must be clear that an opioid-dependent child or student or athlete or employee is inevitably at risk for sudden respiratory death. Therefore, naloxone—and someone who knows how to administer it—must be available in the possible event of rapid respiratory decline.

4. In the situation of long term, or even recent opioid dependency or abuse, all groups must be aware that high-dose buccal buprenorphine (Bunavail, Suboxone, and Zubsolv) is available from certified physicians, and now also from PAs and NPs who are certified to prescribe it for ongoing opioid treatment. Although only a small number of these practitioners are certified, each is now allowed to treat 270 patients (see Resources for access: NAABT).

5. The key to preventing opioid addiction in the first place is for all parents, teachers, coaches, counselors, and employers to be aware of acute injuries, and to find out if the person has been prescribed a short-acting opioid for three to ten days; if yes, to find out when that period expires; and if the injured person is seeking more medication, to suggest a request for low-dose buccal buprenorphine, which can now be prescribed by any provider who has a DEA Schedule III registration.

6. If the at-risk person is older than 17 and, therefore, in direct contact with the doctor for pain relief treatment, the responsible party can give them this guide or suggest to request low-dose buccal buprenorphine if something stronger is needed.

There is a big likelihood that physicians may say they do not prescribe this medication because it requires a special certification. Remind these physicians that buprenorphine is now available in low-dose form under the brand name **Belbuca**. The responsible party should know that any provider who can prescribe Vicodin, Percocet, Oxycontin, and other opioids, may safely prescribe low-dose buprenorphine for pain relief, without the risk of accidental overdose or precipitating withdrawal. Physicians may believe that only pain specialists are capable of prescribing low-dose buprenorphine, which would not be surprising considering the mystery around buprenorphine; but it would be more opportune for the Primary Care Physician (PCP) or orthopedist to prescribe it even before the patient requires a pain specialist.

It is very likely to be confronted by the argument that buprenorphine is also an opioid and might be addictive. An appropriate response would be that while it may lead to mild dependency, it is far less addictive than all other opioids. Buprenorphine is much easier to stop because there is often no withdrawal, or at most very mild withdrawal symptoms. More importantly, it cannot cause an accidental overdose, except in very unusual circumstances when it is combined with another depressant in a very high dose and injected intravenously. If taken in a chronic pain situation, it is also less likely to cause increased neuropathic pain, as noted in the Servick (2016) article and by Pergolizzi et al, 2010.

It really is up to family, friends, teachers, coaches, counselors, and employers to educate those around them, as well as physicians about the safety of buprenorphine and its effectiveness for pain relief in the post-acute phase of an injury. Their actions may ultimately change the statistics linked to those aforementioned 75% first-time heroin users who took narcotic pain pills before switching to heroin.

But why should it be up to parents, coaches, teachers, counselors, and employers to educate physicians?

Many healthcare providers are still under the impression that buprenorphine is too difficult to prescribe without special training. They need to be reminded that any provider with a DEA registration, which is required to prescribe all opioids, can now prescribe buprenorphine too. They also need to be reminded that low doses of buprenorphine are very effective for pain relief and do not cause sudden withdrawal symptoms if someone is on a full agonist opioid. In fact, low dose buprenorphine can actually be combined with other full agonists for increased pain relief (Budd & Raffa, 2005).

While treating and managing addiction is a complex and lifelong process, three simple strategies to decrease sudden death are:

1. Naloxone (Narcan) education and training throughout the country.
2. High dose buprenorphine-naloxone (Bunavail, Suboxone, Zubsolv) for withdrawal and maintenance (MAT).
3. Low dose buprenorphine (Belbuca) for treatment of chronic pain, and hopefully soon for acute pain.

That said, there are three broader strategies to pursue as a nation to end the crisis:

1. Education about opioids.
2. Aggressive, lifelong, treatment of addiction and the funds necessary to do that as well as the willingness of health insurance companies to cover it.
3. The appropriate use of Naloxone, high dose buprenorphine, and low dose buprenorphine by the right people, in the right place, at the right time.

Prince died needlessly. He was dealing with the difficult combination of chronic pain and opioid dependence that has become all too common in our current medical culture. It has now become evident that, to protect his privacy, a friend was getting oxycodone prescriptions filled in his own name and giving them to Prince. The day before he died, an addiction specialist from California was called, so he sent his son to Minnesota carrying high-dose buprenorphine to give to Prince. If he had arrived in time to administer the drug, Prince's opioid receptors would have been satisfied, eliminating the need to turn to the powerful fentanyl that ultimately stopped his respirations and caused his death in that elevator.

Amy died needlessly. If that on-call doctor had not flatly refused to prescribe an opioid to satisfy her opioid receptors, she would not have had to resort to street opioids and ultimately black tar heroin, which stopped her respirations and caused her untimely death in her own bedroom within 30 feet of her parents. A properly educated physician on that Friday night would have known that a very small dose of buccal buprenorphine could have satisfied her opioid receptors and ultimately saved her life.

Rhonda did not die that snowy winter night, because she walked into the emergency room and asked for buprenorphine and not Oxycontin.

In conclusion:
Since the solution really comes down to education about opioids in general and buprenorphine in particular, the most crucial task at hand is to demystify this medication in the minds of the nearly one million physicians in the United States alone. Although this was written for parents, teachers, coaches, and employers, it is my hope that the many excellent physicians, nurse practitioners, and physician assistants in this country who are reluctant to prescribe low dose buccal buprenorphine for chronic pain will see the wisdom in this one safe opioid and realize that there is no mystery attached to it and no difficulty in prescribing it! And further realize that it is Schedule 3, and readily available.

Analogous to there being three phenomena causing the epidemic over the last 20 years, i.e.: the under treatment of pain, Purdue Pharmaceutical, and Xalisco, Mexico, there are three efforts necessary to reverse the number of deaths.

At the risk of repetition and oversimplifying the strategies necessary, they can be boiled down to three words: RESCUE, RECOVERY, and PREVENTION!

RESCUE with Naloxone (Narcan)!

RECOVERY by a lifelong commitment to the treatment of addiction using everything from medication to meditation, along with many more approaches in between (as noted on page 46)!

PREVENTION by choosing low dose buccal buprenorphine as the first opioid of choice if an opioid is deemed necessary, to totally avoid the risk of sudden death, and significantly lower and possibly eliminate the risk of addiction to opioids (chapter 6)!

This epidemic is real, and getting worse, and this is an opportunity to stop this deadly trend!

Appendix A

Strength comparisons of various opioids

Keeping in mind that morphine is the opioid most other opioids are compared to in terms of effectiveness and side effects, the following is a comparison of several commonly prescribed medications, as well as some that have been added to recent batches of heroin. Of those, Codeine is the weakest and Carfentanil the most powerful.

0.003 mg carfentanil
= 0.3 mg fentanyl
= 1 mg buprenorphine
= 7 mg hydromorphone (Dilaudid)
=10 mg oxymorphone (Opana)
= 20 mg oxycodone (Percocet, Roxicet, Oxycontin)
= 20 mg methadone
= 30 mg hydrocodone (Vicodin, Norco)
= 30 mg morphine
= 200 mg codeine.

Appendix B

Dose comparison of low-dose buccal buprenorphine now available for pain (not requiring the 8 hour course) compared to morphine (MsO4).

Higher dose buprenorphine alone or in combination with naloxone (Bunavail, Suboxone, Zubsolv) for addiction treatment has been available since 2003, in doses ranging from two to twelve milligrams (mgs).

Low-dose buprenorphine became available for chronic pain in October, 2016 in doses ranging from 75 to 900 **micrograms (mcgs)**.

The conversions are based on the fact that a microgram (mcg) is 1000th of a milligram (mg) and buprenorphine is approximately 30 times stronger than morphine (MsO4).

Following is a comparison of available doses of low-dose buprenorphine to the equivalent doses of morphine. Doses of other opioids can be extrapolated from Appendix A above. It is worth noting that the highest dose available for pain (900 mcg or 0.9 mg) is just slightly less than half of the lowest dose (2 mg) available for addiction.

900 mcg of buprenorphine = 27 mg of MsO4
750 mcg of buprenorphine = 22.5 mg of MsO4
600 mcg of buprenorphine = 18 mg of MsO4
450 mcg of buprenorphine = 13.5 mg of MsO4
300 mcg of buprenorphine = 9 mg of MsO4
150 mcg of buprenorphine = 4.5 mg of MsO4
75 mcg of buprenorphine = 2.25 mg of MsO4

BIBLIOGRAPHY AND REFERENCES

Azam, A. (2015). Young hands in Mexico feed growing U.S. demand for heroin. *The New York Times*, 8/29/15.

Brick, J., & Erickson, C. (1998). *Drugs, the Brain, and Behavior*. Binghamton, NY: The Haworth Medical Press.

Budd, K., & Collett, B.J. (2003). Old dog—new (ma) trix. *Br. Journal of Anaesth.*, 90:722-24.

Budd,K., & Raffa, R., (2005). *Buprenorphine–The Unique Opioid Analgesic*. New York, NY and Stuttgart, Germany. Thieme Verlag.

Campos-Outcalt, D. (2016). Opioids for chronic pain: The CDC's 12 recommendations. *The Journal of Family Practice*, 65(12):906-909.

Cicero, T.J., et al. (2014). The changing face of heroin use in the U.S: a retrospective analysis of the past 50 years. *JAMA Psychiatry*, 71(7):821-6.

Clinical Guidelines for the Treatment of Opioid Addiction. Treatment Improvement Protocol (TIP) Series, No. 40. DHHS Pub #04-3939, Rockville, MD; 2004.

Courtwright, D.T. (1982 & 2001). *Dark Paradise: A History of Opiate Addiction in America*. Cambridge, MA and London, UK: Harvard University Press.

Cowan, et al. (1977). Agonist and antagonist properties of buprenorphine, a new antinociceptive agent. *Br. J. Pharmacol*, 60:537-545.

Dahan, A., et al. (2006). Buprenorphine induces ceiling in respiratory depression but not in analgesia *Br. J. Anaesth.*, 96(5):627-32, (2006).

Daitch, D., et al. (2014). Conversion from high-dose full-opioid agonists to sublingual buprenorphine reduces pain scores and improves quality of Life for chronic pain patients. *Pain Medicine*, 15:2087-2094.

Dowell, D., Haegerich, T.M., & Chou, R. (2016). *CDC Guideline for Prescribing Opioids for Chronic Pain— United States*, 65:1-49.

Erickson, C. (2007). *The Science of Addiction*. New York, NY: W.W. Norton Co.

Fernandez, H. (1998). *Heroin*. Center City, MN: Hazelden.

Gable, R.S., (2004). Comparison of acute lethal toxicity of commonly abused psychoactive substances. *NCBI.* 99(6):686-96 [doi:10.1111/j.1360-0443.2004.00744.x]

Ingraham, C. (2016). CDC data shows heroin deaths surpass gun homicides for the first time. *The Washington Post*, 12/8/16.

Jasinski, D., et al. (1978). Human pharmacology and abuse potential of the analgesic buprenorphine, *NCBI. Arch. Gen. Psychiatry*, 35:501-516.

Kintz, P. & Marquet, P. (1984). *Buprenorphine Therapy of Opiate Addiction*. Totowa, NJ: Humana Press.

Lembke, A. (2016). *Drug Dealer, MD*. Baltimore, MD: Johns Hopkins University Press.

Lopez, G. (2017). *Vox.*

Lopez, G. (2018). Surgeon General report. Vox.

Marteau, D., et al. (2015). The relative risk of fatal poisoning by methadone or buprenorphine within the wider population of England and Wales. *BMJ Open*, 5(5): e007629.

Martell, B.A., et al. (2007). Systematic review: opioid treatment for chronic back pain: prevalence, efficacy, and association with addiction. *Ann. Internal Med.*, 146(2):116-27.

Mercadante, S., et al. (2006). Safety and effectiveness of IV morphine for episodic breakthrough pain in patients receiving transdermal Buprenorphine. *J. Pain Management*, 32 (2):175-9.

Morbidity and Mortality Weekly Report (MMWR) by Centers for Disease Control and Prevention. 1600 Clifton Rd., Atlanta, GA.

National Safety Council Survey (2017).

Nelson, S. *USA Today*, 8/25/16.

Paone, D., et al. (2015). Buprenorphine infrequently found in fatal overdose in NYC. *Drug Alcohol Depend.* 155:298-301.

Pergolizzi, J., et al. (2010). Current knowledge of buprenorphine and its unique pharmacological profile. *NCBI*, 10(5)428-450. doi: 10.1111/j.1533-2500.2010.00378.x.

Pergolizzi, J., et al. (2016). Management of moderate to severe chronic low back pain with buprenorphine buccal film using novel bioerodible mucoadhesive Technology. *J. Pain Res.* 9:909-916.

Portenoy R.K., & Foley K.M. (1986). Chronic use of opioid analgesics in non-malignant pain: report of 38 cases. *PAIN,* 25(2): 171-186.

Physicians for Responsible Opioid Prescribing (PROP) Website, retrieved from www.supportprop.org. Portenoy video in Educational Materials, CME (Resources).

Quinones, S. (2015). *Dreamland, The True Tale of America's Opiate Crisis.* New York, NY: Bloomsbury Press.

Servick, K. (2016). Why painkillers sometimes make pain worse. *SCIENCE,*

Stein, B.D., et al. (2016). Physician capacity to treat opioid use disorder with buprenorphine-assisted treatment. *JAMA,* 316:1211-1212.

Szalavitz, M. (2015). *Unbroken Brain.* New York, NY: St. Martin's Press.

Tallarida, R.J. (2000). *Drug Synergism and Dose-Effect Data Analysis.* Boca Raton, FL: Chapman & Hall/CRC.

Werner, A. (2017). Did NFL doctors and trainers push powerful painkillers on players? *CBS News,* 3/10/17.

RESOURCES

National Alliance and Advocates for
Buprenorphine Treatment (NAABT) to access
names of certified physicians

Naloxone- National Institute on Drug Abuse
(NIDA) website.

Substance Abuse and Mental Health Services
Administration (SAMHSA) publication, 3/03/16 on
Naloxone.

The Atlantic, *The Fight for the Overdose Drug*,
December, 2014.

www.bdsi.com for information on low dose
buccal buprenorphine.

www.thefix.com

Glossary of Terms:

AED
Automated External Defibrillator

Agonist
An agonist is an activator or a stimulus. It can be an internal chemical or hormone, such as an endorphin. It can also be an external chemical or drug such as morphine. Agonists are either full or partial. Full agonists can reach their full potential if enough is given, i.e. if enough heroin is taken, it will reach its full potential and stop respirations. Partial agonists do not reach full potential for some of their effects, but they will plateau and not go higher.

Belbuca
The current brand of low dose buccal buprenorphine.

Buccal
The inside of the cheek.

CARA
Comprehensive Addiction and Recovery Act

CDC
Centers for Disease Control

CNS
Central Nervous System

CPR
Cardiopulmonary Resuscitation

DATA 2000
Drug Addiction Treatment Act of 2000

DEA
Drug Enforcement Administration

FDA
Food and Drug Administration

Gram
A metric unit of weight equal to .04 ounces.

HC
Hydrocodone

IV
Intravenous (injected directly into a vein)

Microgram (mcg)
.001 (one thousandth) of a milligram (mg)

Milligram (mg)
.001 (one thousandth) of a gram (gm)

MAT
Medication Assisted Treatment

MsO4
Morphine Sulfate

NIH
National Institutes of Health

NP
Nurse Practitioner

OC
Oxycodone

Opium
Raw substance extracted from the pulp of the poppy plant.

Opiates
Extracted from opium.

Opioids
Synthesized from opiates.

Oxycontin
Long acting, sustained release form of oxycodone.

PA
Physician's Assistant

PCP
Primary Care Provider

Percocet
One of the brand names of oxycodone combined with acetaminophen (Tylenol).

Receptor
A receptor is a series of amino acids and/or proteins that exist in the brain, and attract agonists in such a way that it becomes activated and causes a physiological response in the brain and/or body.

SQ
Subcutaneous (injected under the skin).

Sublingual
Under the tongue.

Vicodin
One of the brand names of hydrocodone combined with acetaminophen (Tylenol).

INDEX

A

addiction 1, 5, 11, 15, 19, 27, 34, 46, 54
agonist 15, 34
alcohol 7, 13, 21
antagonist 8, 15, 34
automated external defibrillator (AED) 22, 44

B

Baker, Chet 7
Belbuca 45, 48, 50
Belushi, John 7
benzodiazepine 13, 21, 36
black tar heroin 6, 31, 45, 51
Bunavail 37, 41, 44, 47, 50, 54
buprenorphine 4, 20, 25, 33, 39, 43, 48, 53, 54

C

carfentanil 17, 19, 53
CDC 2, 5, 45
codeine 16, 53
Comprehensive Addiction and Recovery Act (CARA) 26
Controlled Substance Act 25
CPR 22, 44

D

Dark Paradise 2, 5, 11, 24
DATA 2000 25, 26
DEA 25, 39, 47
depressants 9, 13
Dilaudid 17, 46, 53
Dreamland 31, 46
Drug Dealer, MD 46

E

endorphins 12

F

FDA 2, 36, 40, 45
fentanyl 7, 17, 47, 50, 53
Friedman, Michael 30
full agonist 15, 19, 35, 40, 49

G

Goldenheim, Paul 30

H

Harrison Narcotics Act 24
heroin 1, 5, 14, 15, 18, 23, 27, 31, 33, 39, 45, 49, 53
Hoffman, Philip Seymour 7, 46
Holiday, Billie 7
hydrocodone 17, 29, 46, 53
hydromorphone 17, 46, 53

I

intravenous 35, 49

J

Jick, Hershel 28
Joplin, Janis 7

L

Lembke, Anna MD 11, 46
Lewis, John W 34
Lortab 17

M

medication assisted treatment 46
Medication Assisted Treatment 43
methadone 17, 24, 37, 44, 53
microgram 54
milligram 54
morphine 8, 15, 19, 24, 27, 34, 41, 53, 54

N

naloxone 4, 19, 22, 36, 43, 50, 52, 54
naltrexone 44
Narcan 19, 22, 50, 52
Narcotics Farm 34
National Safety Council Survey 46
Nayarit 31
NFL 6
Norco 17, 53
nurse practitioner 26, 46, 51

O

opiate 16, 17, 28
opioid 1, 5, 12, 15, 19, 24, 27, 33, 38, 43, 50, 53, 54
opium 1, 5, 8, 16, 24, 27, 31
oxycodone 17, 29, 46, 50, 53
Oxycontin 6, 17, 29, 38, 41, 48, 51, 53

P

Parker, Charlie 7
partial agonist 15, 34, 43
Percocet 6, 17, 41, 43, 46, 48, 53
Portenoy, Russel MD 28
Prince 7, 19, 50
PROP 29
Purdue Pharmaceutical 29, 51
Pure Food and Drug Act 24

Q

Quinones, Sam 31, 46

R

receptor 12, 15, 22, 37, 40, 44, 50
Reckitt-Coleman 34
relaxers 13

S

Saunders, Cicely 27
stimulant 9, 13, 21
subcutaneous 35
sublingual 35, 38
sudden death 1, 5, 8, 21, 27, 36, 43, 46, 49, 52

ACKNOWLEDGEMENTS

I am grateful to all the people who motivated me to complete this project.

Lane Wagaman, Ed.D, Trudi Taylor, Ph.D, Helena Trangata, Brenda and Lyle Kitt, Frances O'Halloran, Bob Thompson, Mukesh Kamdar, MD, Leeza Steindorf, Linda DelMonaco Willard, Suzana McCalley, Jone van Rees, Belinda Nicoll, Jason Bohde, Jacob Buckmaster, Abigail Mancini, my Monday writing group, and most recently, Mae and Eleanor.

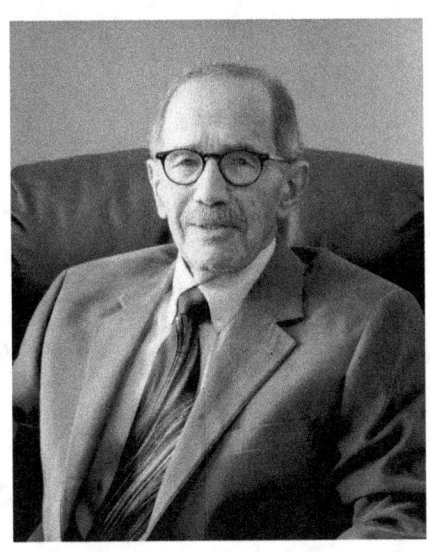

After graduating from medical school and completing a family practice residency, Dr. Mancini practiced family medicine in Washington, DC and Rochester, NY. Board certified in Family Medicine and Addiction Medicine, the last 10 years of his practice were combined with specific care in Addiction Medicine, primarily for opioid-dependent people.

In addition to his medical license, Dr. Mancini has acquired a Masters Degree in Medical Education while on the faculty at the University of Rochester. Dr. Mancini was a Clinical Associate Professor of Family Medicine at the University of Rochester School of Medicine and Dentistry, and served as Chief of Family Practice at Rochester General Hospital. He is currently the president of SOON (Stop Opioid Overdose Now), a non-profit opioid education foundation.

Dr. Mancini can be reached at:
josephcmancini@gmail.com or (585) 645-9245
for speaking engagements or questions.